HANNAH SHARP

Childbirth On Your Terms

Tips to Have a Quick, Easy, Natural Labor and Delivery

This book was professionally typeset on Reedsy.
Find out more at reedsy.com

Contents

1

Introduction

In this book, you will learn several ways to induce labor naturally and how to cope with the pain of labor and delivery. Whether this is your first baby or a subsequent pregnancy, these things may help you have a quick, natural labor and delivery. As a disclaimer: this is not medical advice, and you should always discuss things with your doctor before you try to induce labor at home. These things worked for me, but that does not mean they will work for you or are safe for you and your pregnancy. Once again, please discuss this with your healthcare provider.

Everli's Birth Story

I want to start my book by telling you the story of my labor and delivery with my first child. It was the most exciting experience, and I almost crave doing it again.

When I got pregnant the first time, I was scared and excited. Throughout my pregnancy, I thought about the finish line often. The birth, the inevitable part, and the most exciting part is when you finally get to be done with nausea and pain, and you get to meet your baby. My first birth was the most amazing experience I could have ever asked for, everything went as planned, and the people around me were amazing. I knew I wanted to have a natural birth and I knew I wanted to do anything in my power not to have an induction. I had talked with many friends and family members that had inductions and it was extra painful and took a very long time. At 34 weeks, my doctor had already brought up induction, to say it scared me is an understatement. My husband was my saving grace and was on my side for all of it. He supported me in my decision to have a natural birth and helped me without giving in. Without him, I don't know if I could have done it.

During my pregnancy I educated myself on the many ways to go into labor naturally, I tried most of them but not all. At 38 weeks pregnant the baby is considered full-term, so at that time I started doing things to cause labor in order to avoid induction. At 39 weeks I was already dilated to a 3 and my doctor did a membrane sweep. Three days later, the evening before my due date, I started having contractions or what I thought might be real contractions. I called the hospital and talked with a nurse, she told me to go to bed and see if anything progressed. Lo and behold, my contractions had stopped and I got a full night's rest.

The day of my due date arrived, I had my husband take a photo of me, as I had been doing every week. I put an eviction notice on the photo as a joke. My husband and I did some running around and by noon, I started having contractions again. They started very slow but continued to increase in length and strength. (Another thing I knew I wanted was to labor as long as possible in the comfort of my own home.) By 5 pm, my contractions had ramped-up to the point that I couldn't talk through them, so I started tracking them with an app on my phone. My husband made me a steak dinner to make sure I had the strength for the journey we were about to embark on. After about 45 minutes of tracking my contractions following the 5:1:1 rule, my husband started to get worried and wanted to go to the hospital. We packed up the last of our things and headed 20 minutes to Madras, Oregon.

Once we got to the hospital it started snowing pretty intensely, the nurses checked me and I was only 4 centimeters dilated. Since it was snowing and I was having consistently strong contractions they said they were going to keep me for two hours and monitor my progression. They also stated I probably wasn't going to have the baby tonight. 45 minutes later, I had a big contraction and felt the big pop of my water breaking. I told my husband that I thought my water had just broken, and he told me we should probably call the nurse. The nurse checked and confirmed my water had broken; she told me that it earned me a full admission, but I probably still wouldn't have my baby tonight.

After my water had broken, my contractions intensified tenfold. I was in the most pain of my life but in between my contractions, I could breathe and get a bit of a break to prepare for the next contraction. My labor progressed so quickly that the nurses were in complete shock. I remember when my doctor got there and sat in my room, checking me every once in a while to see if the baby was crowning. When it came to pushing, it was the hardest work my body had ever done. (Looking back I would rather labor than have that final push) 45 minutes of pushing and I didn't know if I could do it anymore. My contraction stopped and I completely stopped pushing, I looked my doctor straight in the eye and told her I refused to push again. She told me I had no choice. One more push and my baby girl was in my arms.

Everli Jo was born on her due date, February 12th, 2021, at 10:19 p.m. She came into the world like a rocket and hasn't stopped moving since.

I would consider my labor to have been 6 hours. My nurses and doctor told me that it was not at all normal to have a baby on their due date and have your first baby so fast. I like to think that the things I did through and towards the end of my pregnancy had something to do with having a successful natural birth.

2

Understanding Natural Birth

Natural birth refers to the process of giving birth without the assistance of pain medication, allowing the body to follow its natural course. There are various options available to women who wish to have a natural birth, including hospital births, home births, or birth center deliveries. It's important to note that even though natural birth is a safe and fulfilling experience for many women, there is always a possibility of complications. Therefore, some women choose to have their natural birth in a hospital, where they can receive expert medical care from their trusted healthcare provider, as I did.

It's common for individuals who opt for a natural birth to choose to do so in the comfort of their own homes. However, it's worth noting that giving birth naturally is also achievable in a hospital setting. Unfortunately, some individuals may face resistance from their obstetricians, who may attempt to persuade them to undergo inductions or even cesarean sections.

The benefits of having a natural labor and delivery are:

- Labor and delivery are often faster
- More efficient pushing
- Less risk of tearing
- Less pain after delivery
- Lower chance of a Caesarian section
- Faster recovery time
- Baby is more alert and more apt to breastfeeding

Having a natural birth can give you a more empowered state of mind. After I gave birth naturally, I felt like I could do anything! Those who once told me I couldn't do it or called me crazy no longer had any hold on me.

The medications given during labor have been shown to affect the baby as well. It can cause the mother to have lower than normal blood pressure, which lowers the amount of oxygen going to the baby. When the baby gets an oxygen deficiency, it can cause their heart rate to drop, in turn making it more likely to have a C-section.

Mothers generally feel much better following right after a natural birth, most likely due to the rush of endorphins. Endorphins are released when you are stressed or in pain. They block the nerve cells receiving the pain. Endorphins and dopamine work together to make you feel better. Dopamine is the happiness hormone; it is released when we eat something delicious or do something fun. So, when we are in a large amount of pain with childbirth, endorphins are released to block the nerves from feeling pain, and then dopamine is released to make us feel joy. This may be why you hear about women who have had natural deliveries, smiling and even giggling during the most painful parts of childbirth.

Some people think it is crazy that women choose to endure childbirth over and over again, even though the pain is equivalent to breaking 20 bones all at the same time. But our bodies are made to do this. The chemicals in our brains protect us from all the pain and make us feel the most joy we could imagine, almost craving the feeling again.

Natural birth is unlike anything you will ever experience, and it's incredible to feel and see what your body was designed to do. You will feel more empowered and enriched in what you didn't know you were capable of. You were born for this, and you can do this.

3

Your Birth Plan

I will not show you how to create a written birth plan; this is more about the essentials of having a successful birth. Don't get me wrong, a written birth plan is very valuable to give to your doctor and nurses to establish how you would like your birth to go and to set expectations for yourself. It can also answer a lot of the questions your medical staff might have if you are like me and are already in labor when you arrive at the hospital. It can be challenging to compile thoughts and discussions when you are in labor.

While you are pregnant, whether for the first time or anytime after that, you should always try to educate yourself. Things in the medical world are constantly changing. New discoveries arise, and new medications and practices come into the hospitals. You should always ask your doctors and nurses questions about their practices and, if it's the same doctor, if there is anything they would do differently. The power of education can help ease your anxiety and fear. It can be much easier when you know what to expect.

When I was pregnant with my first, I watched all the birth preparation videos so I knew what to expect. I also did my own research about almost everything, from what I should take to the hospital to what choices I had. Since you have bought this book, you are already on the right track! Yay!

Some of the things you should educate yourself on are your pain management options, what your partner can do for you in labor, and what kind of environment you want to have. These things can be essential when you are in labor and will help you make the best decisions for yourself.

Talk with your doctor and healthcare team about their different pain management options; hospitals and even doctors have different pain management options they like to use. While I was in labor, I did get one dose of a narcotic; it took a bit of the edge off and helped me regain my thoughts. In my mind, I would say I had a successful natural birth. I had a bit of help, but I did not get an epidural, so for me, that was a win. Others might disagree and say that since I had medication to help ease my pain, it could not be considered a natural birth. Well, I am here to say that all that matters is how I see my birth as a win. If you choose to get pain medication of any kind, you will not lose; the actual win is a healthy baby and a healthy mom.

Another thing you should educate yourself on (and maybe your partner) is how your partner can help you in labor. There are many ways they can help manage your pain, be your voice, or just be a comforting presence in the room. We were still in the middle of a COVID-19 lock down when I had my daughter. Before COVID, I imagined having my mom, mother-in-law, and maybe my sister in the room. I never imagined not having the opportunity to kick anyone out. Looking back, I wouldn't have it any other way. It was so calm and comforting having just my husband, the one who had been standing by my side the whole time. The one who knew I could do it without faltering. My biggest mistake was not showing him how to do the massages that could help me in labor.

Talk to your partner about your goals and how they can support you, whether physical touch or reminding you that you can do this. Your partner will want to be involved even if they haven't told you specifically. A good thing to remember is you are going to be enduring the most pain you have ever felt, and you do not know what you might want during that time. Understanding that your wants and needs may change during labor will help your partner know they are not doing anything wrong when you yell at them or smack them away. (Trust me, that happens.)

Your partner can also be a way to provide you with a supportive environment. If they understand what you want, then they can make it happen. Some things people don't think of when it comes to having an excellent birthing environment are lighting, sound, and smell. Much like how a baby likes a dark room, white noise, and lavender to calm themselves to sleep, those things can help calm your mind while you are in pain. Choosing low lighting or having some twinkle lights to calm your senses can help focus your energy. Most of the mothers I have talked with who had natural births had their babies at night. The dimness of the night can help your body and mind relax, releasing more oxytocin, which is the hormone that helps with contractions.

Music or white noise can drown out some of the background noise of your healthcare team talking or, in my case, the TV that accidentally got left on. You might want something relaxing to help you breathe through your contractions or music to help you remember how strong you are and what awaits you. Some songs I had on my playlist were:

- Firework by Katy Perry
- Haven't Met You Yet by Michael Buble
- Hurts So Good by Astrid S
- I won't give up by Jason Mraz
- I am Woman by Emmy meli

These are just a few that I listened to; after you get into the groove of labor, sometimes it all fades into the background.

Certain smells, such as lavender, chamomile, sandalwood, and clary sage, also help calm you. There are several other scents for stress relief you can try as well. Essential oils are the most acceptable form of these to use in hospitals. The great thing about using essential oils is you can use them in many ways: massage oil, added to a bath, or just a roll-on form that you can put on your wrist to smell.

4

Body Preparations

Your body is about to go through the most challenging job you ever have to do. I know, no duh, right, but truly understanding and connecting with your body is crucial. Now, you might be thinking, "Connect with my body? How can I get more connected to something already connected to me?" Those are very good questions. Connecting to your body is more about connecting your mind with your physical self, feeling every part of your body, feeling your baby, and listening to what your body is trying to tell you. Many of us get so busy with the day-to-day that we don't listen to what our body is genuinely trying to say to us, such as where the pain is, what we should do to help with the pain, and what nourishment we need. All these things can be heard when you stop and listen.

Try sitting in silence and really think about what your body is trying to tell you. Similar to meditating, but you don't have to think about something special or listen to anyone guiding you through the process. There are videos out there you can follow if you need more guidance. I have found it helpful to listen to one video and then do it on my own after that. Find somewhere comfortable to sit or lie down and think

12

about every part of your body, truly feeling it. Starting from your head, arms, and hands, then your legs and feet, feeling your breath and your heartbeat and noting all your feelings, good or bad. Finally, focus on your stomach and your baby, feel where the baby is and how the baby is moving, and focus on your pelvis and your uterus and how it is going to give you this beautiful baby soon. Doing this will help you truly start to connect with your body. Do this several times throughout your pregnancy. Just feel what your body and baby are telling you and get connected. When you are in labor, connecting with your body will be very important for a natural birth. Your body will tell you what positions to get into to help with the pain and what you have to do to get your baby out.

Walking is also a way to prepare your body. While walking has many benefits on its own, during pregnancy, it can help you stay active and keep your body healthy. I started walking right away during my pregnancy, although I found out I was pregnant in June, so it was the perfect weather for walking my dogs and getting my little niece out of the house. If you already have an exercise routine, that's great! Stick with it throughout your pregnancy. If you were doing it before, such as weight lifting or CrossFit, keep doing it throughout your pregnancy while listening to your body and toning it back when needed. If you are like me and did not exercise regularly before your pregnancy, walking for 20-30 minutes daily is a simple way to prepare your body for the main workout of birth. Walking will help reduce the risk of gestational diabetes and help keep the weight gain under control. It can also help boost your mood and get better sleep. Further along in your pregnancy, walking can help with back and pelvic pain, moving the baby into a more comfortable position for you. When you get right close to your due date, walking can also help move the baby's head down into your pelvis and get it into the proper position to prepare for labor.

Walking and other types of exercise can be hard on your joints in pregnancy, especially your hips. Bouncing on a yoga ball can help release some of the pressure on your hips, pelvis, and tailbone. There are various ways to use a yoga ball: bouncing, hip circles, lying over it to stretch your arms, or lying over it backward to stretch your lower back. This can also help get the baby into an optimal position and help move the baby down into your pelvic floor as it opens and loosens up. During labor, the ball can be used if you are on all fours; you can drape your arms over it and rest your head. You can also put your leg into a lunge to help open up your pelvis even more, making your contractions more effective.

Body preparations can also take place outside of your body. If one of your worries is about vaginal tearing, then doing a perineum massage and stretches can help with that. I also partnered this with evening primrose oil, which can help with cervical ripening and effacement. Waiting to start the evening primrose oil until 38 weeks is strongly recommended as it can cause premature birth, and we don't want that! The perineum is the area between your vulva and anus and is where women most tend to tear during delivery. I did not know there were tools by Frida Mom, and Perimom that you can use to do these stretches on your own without struggling. I did these stretches independently, which can be difficult with a large belly. When I got the courage to ask my husband to help, it boosted not only the efficiency of the massage but also the intimacy and trust between us. To do the massage and stretches, make sure you have clean hands and use oil to reduce the friction; you can use coconut or olive oil or any nonsynthetic lubricant or oil. Insert your thumbs slightly into the opening of the vagina, and apply pressure to the bottom wall of the vagina toward your anus; hold this for about 30-60 seconds. You should feel a slight burning sensation; give yourself a slight break, then stretch again for another 30-60 seconds, repeating for about 2 minutes. Then, to massage, move your thumbs in a U-shape along the sides and bottom wall; the entire massage should only take about 5 minutes.

During the stretches and massage, you should stay relaxed, both physically and mentally. This is a great time to practice breathing through pain in that area and conditioning yourself to prepare for the ring of fire. If you have not heard of the term "ring of fire," it refers to the burning sensation that occurs when the largest part of the baby's head is being delivered.

The evening primrose oil that I mentioned before can be used to soften and thin your cervix. Having an unripe cervix can lead to prolonged labor and increase the chances of having medical intervention. It will not cause contractions but can take some of the load off in early labor, making for quicker active labor. Softening and effacement of the cervix can cause dilation without contractions before active labor. I was dilated to 3 cm four days prior to going into actual labor. There are several ways you can take evening primrose oil, either by mouth or inserted into the vagina right up next to the cervix. I did both of these starting at 38 weeks, take one capsule by mouth three times a day, and at night, poke a hole in the capsule with a needle and insert into the vagina. It will dissolve overnight by doing all the work while you sleep. I suggest putting a panty liner on if you are worried about oil stains.

The best thing to get labor going is The Miles Circuit. I recommend this to all of my friends and family who want to go into labor naturally and avoid induction. The circuit is a set of positions to help get labor going if it has stalled or slowed, and it can help with turning or getting the baby in the optimal position for delivery. It was created by Sharon Muza, CD(CONA), LCCE, DONA Approved Birth Doula Trainer, and

Megan Miles, a birth doula, when they were helping a mother to get her labor to progress. There are three positions: Open Knee Chest, starting in cat/cow pose on all fours, then drop your chest to the floor or bed; you can also do an advanced version and have your knees up on a couch and lower your chest to the floor, you can put some pillows on the floor to keep yourself comfortable. Try to stay in this position for 30 minutes if you can. The second position is exaggerated side lying; lay on your side, bend, and put your top leg as high as possible with many pillows or a peanut ball, keep your bottom leg straight, and roll onto your belly as much as possible. If you end up falling asleep in this position, great; if not, try to stay in this position for at least 30 minutes. The last position is what I like to call the Captain Morgan pose: get a step stool and put one foot up, and you can do this out in front of you or to the side. Try to square up your hips and not lean into it. The key is being asymmetrical and opening your pelvis. Stay in this position for 30 minutes; I like to switch legs halfway through. While in the last pose, you can also work on your breathing and relax. Think about moving your baby down into your pelvis, as you breathe out, tighten your muscles, and slightly push your baby down, you should feel the pressure of the baby pushing down into your pelvis.

I also liked to help push my baby into my pelvis whenever I went to the bathroom. The toilet has also been called the dilation station because our bodies are used to relaxing and letting everything go down and out. Many people have had their babies on the toilet, both on accident and on purpose. It is a beneficial tool both before labor and in labor.

Remember, the last couple of body preparations I mentioned should not be done until you are considered full-term, 37-38 weeks a long. Other than connecting with your body and walking (which should be done during your entire pregnancy), perineum massage, evening primrose oil, and the miles circuit have the possibility of sending you into labor, so you want to make sure your baby is ready and fully baked before attempting these.

5

Coping With Contactions

When your body starts going into labor, one of the best things you can do to ease your anxiety is to know what's to come. There are four stages of labor: early labor, active labor, pushing or delivery of your baby, and then the delivery of your placenta. I will only be talking about the first three in this book. Early labor is generally quite easy and unpredictable; these contractions are mild and irregular. During this time, you might experience losing your mucus plug, a thick layer of mucus covering your cervix to help protect your baby. Early labor can last anywhere from a couple of days to only several hours. To cope through these contractions, you can take a bath, have your partner give you a massage, go for a walk, or just change positions. These contractions can be very sporadic or don't get stronger, longer, or closer together. Get as much rest as you can if you feel early labor is starting because you are just at the beginning of your marathon.

Active labor is what everyone thinks about when you say that you are in labor. This stage of labor starts when your contractions get stronger, longer, and closer together. A good rule of thumb is the 511 rule: when your contractions are five minutes apart, lasting one minute, and this continues for one hour, this is also when they will usually tell you to head to the hospital. Active labor can be the most exhausting part of the process as your body does the most work during this time. Your contractions are pushing your baby down into the birthing canal, and typically, this is when your cervix is dilating from about 6 centimeters to 10 centimeters. This will be the time to remember your breathing and do low moans and groans as you need to. A lower octave will help you stay focused and not exhaust more energy during contractions. Between contractions, try to relax and regroup your mind; the best thing you can do is just let go of the last contraction and let go of everything around you.

To manage your pain during this time, you can:

- Take a bath or shower
- Have your partner give you a massage between contractions or provide you with counter pressure in your hips and lower back
- Listen to soothing or encouraging music
- Use aroma therapy to stay calm and focused
- Change positions as your body tells you to

A bath will take some pressure off your back and give you the warmth and comfort to relax during your labor. Water can be very comforting; if you don't prefer baths, a shower with your partner gives you a massage or counter pressure. Counter pressure helps relieve back pain and back labor.

There are several types of counter pressure, such as hip squeeze and sacral pressure. The hip squeeze is just what you imagine: have your partner put the heel of their hands on each hip with their fingers pointing up and squeezing together. For the sacral counter pressure, have your partner put their whole hand on that sacrum bone and hold firm pressure. Both of these measures should be done starting when your contraction begins and continuing through the entirety of the contraction. Practicing these with your partner while you are pregnant will help you know the proper position and amount of pressure you will need. Also, during your contractions, remember to communicate if you need more or less pressure or if you need their hands to be positioned somewhere else. These counter pressures can be very difficult for your partner, so if you have other support, that can take over for a little while if it is helping you cope with your contractions.

Listening to music and using aroma therapy can help keep your mind and body calm during labor. Whether in the hospital or at home, a lot will be going on around you. So, staying in the zone and staying connected to your body during this time will be very important. Music can help you tune almost everything around you out, and it can also help encourage you to keep pushing through your labor. As Gary Allen says, every storm runs out of rain; the end will come, you just have to get through the little bit of storm.

All those connecting with your body exercises and times when you were listening to what your body is trying to tell you will come into play here. From this point to the point that your baby arrives, your body will be telling you how to change your position to help you with pain and help move your baby into this world faster. It is very important to stay calm and listen to your instincts on how your body needs to be to bring your baby to you. Women have been giving birth for thousands of years, and you have more knowledge than they did back then; trusting your instincts will be essential. Your body was made to have this baby, and you are trusting your body and your baby will be the key to a successful natural birth.

Once it becomes time to push, you are at the final stretch, and your baby is almost in your arms. Talk with your doctor and healthcare team about the different positions in which you can give birth to your baby. Sometimes, your body will tell you to give birth standing, squatting, or lying down, and your doctors can accommodate those positions.

You should wait until you have an undeniable urge. If this is your first delivery, it might feel like you have been pushing for a long time during your contractions. I know I did. When my nurse asked if I was feeling the urge to push, I told her I thought I might have already been doing that. But you will know a difference when it comes to the actual pushing. This will help with less pushing time and less chances of tearing. While pushing, you might hear your healthcare team tell you to hold your breath and bear down. This can be very effective, but sometimes you just can't hold your breath that long; you have also been practicing dealing with pain through breathing. Listen to your body, and you can also breathe the baby out. Take a big breath in right before you start, and slowly release your breath while pushing your baby down and out. The relief will be overwhelming when your baby is finally in your arms. There's a saying that labor is the most painful experience that is also quickest forgotten.

6

Feeling Empowered By Your Birth

It is not the end of your journey after you have your beautiful baby in your arms. Birth can tremendously affect your self-esteem, how you look at the world, and how you handle things to come. Whether you have a natural birth or receive medication throughout the process, it is essential to remember to give yourself some grace. You just went through something people can't even imagine. Bringing life into this world is an incredible accomplishment, and your body's remarkable strength and resilience made it possible.

Your body has changed, with stretch marks, loose skin, and maybe new scars. It can be hard to live up to the expectations society or loved ones put on us. After giving birth, you should focus on physical healing and connecting with your newborn. The expectations are highly unrealistic and you should give yourself some grace for not "bouncing back."

This book is all about how to give birth naturally, but I want to tell you the story of my second labor and delivery to remind everyone that sometimes things do not go as planned, and that is okay.

I got pregnant with my son in December 2022, and I was more excited about giving birth again than I was about being pregnant. Throughout my pregnancy, I had absolutely no complications. The baby and I were healthy and doing great. Six weeks prior to my due date, I woke up to the feeling that the baby was pushing on my bladder, and I thought I was going to pee the bed. I stood up out of bed, and there was a large rush of fluid in my mind, I had just peed my pants. I took a shower to wash off, and my husband peeked his head into the shower to see if I was okay. While I was in the shower I had this thought that maybe my water had broken. I live an hour and a half away from the hospital, and we had plans that day, so I didn't want to inconvenience anyone if I just peed my pants, so I got out of the shower and put a pad on. My husband and I were getting things ready to go to the event we had planned, and I kept getting small releases of fluid that just didn't feel right.

My husband told me to drop everything, and we were headed to the hospital. During our drive, I started to get worried as I could feel some contractions start up, but it was too early. I didn't even get to do any of my body preparations, I didn't have my bags packed or the car seat installed.

We got to the hospital, and the nurses confirmed that my waters had partially broken and I was, in fact, going into labor. It was utterly unknown how this happened or what might have caused it. In Madras, Oregon, where I had given birth to my daughter, there is not a NICU facility. This means that I would have to give birth in Bend, Oregon. To say I was upset was an understatement, but I wasn't about ready to be stuck in Madras while my son was flown to the NICU.

Since my labor and delivery were so quick with my first, the healthcare team was worried I would not make it to Bend before I gave birth.

(Your subsequent labors tend to go quicker as your body has done it before and knows what to do.) They gave me a dose of medication to stop my contractions while we were waiting for the ambulance to arrive. The ambulance took longer than expected, so they had to give me another dose of that medication to stop my contractions when they finally arrived. My husband had to follow the ambulance to Bend in our car, so we were not stranded without any mode of transportation.

Once we arrived at the Bend hospital, things tended to take a turn for the worse. They had to restart my labor as the medication to stall my labor stopped it completely. I had not educated myself on any of this, so my anxiety was through the roof, and I was not prepared to advocate for myself. I knew one thing: I did not want pitocin. Pitocin is a synthetic version of the hormone oxytocin. Oxytocin is responsible for causing your uterus to contract. It can become dangerous to both the mother and the baby when your uterus is forced to contract too hard and too fast. This can cause uterine rupture, postpartum hemorrhage and can put an immense amount of pressure on the baby, restricting blood flow to the brain and causing brain damage to the baby.

After explaining this to the doctor, we settled on starting Cervidil. Cervidil is used to ripen the cervix and prepare it for dilation. Cervidil can be given orally, through an IV, or vaginally. Since my waters had already broken, my baby and I were at an increased risk for infection, eliminating the ability to receive it vaginally. Several rounds of Cervidil and 24 hours later by, contractions had increased in strength, but I could not feel them at all, and my labor was still stalling out.

My healthcare team expressed that they do not want me to go longer than 48 hours with my water broken as the risk of infection increases after that amount of time. We tried massage, the miles circuit, the birthing ball, and many other things to get my labor progressing naturally, but nothing was working. We inevitably had to resort to Pitocin and almost everything I was afraid of happened. During the night, my nurses had to increase and decrease the amount of Pitocin several times as my baby's heart rate kept dropping, and the contractions were still not getting strong enough for me to feel them.

At 48 hours of my water being broken, the third doctor that I had came into my room and told me it was time for my worst nightmare, a C-Section. We had tried everything in our power to help my little boy make his way into the world, and everything failed. I called my mom and broke down for the first time. All I ever wanted was to feel the power of giving birth to my child vaginally, and it felt like it was being ripped from my fingertips.

As I was being wheeled into the operating room, I was emotionally numb. I had asked if I could wear sterile gloves and help deliver my baby, but they denied my request. I got a spinal block and they put a sheet to block my view. The anesthesiologist told me I could open the sheet window to see my baby after he was born. After they made the incision and pulled the baby out, they forgot to pull the window open, so I ripped it open and yelled I want to see! They showed me my boy and pushed him up against the plastic so I could kiss him through the lining. Then, off he went to the NICU team. He had a hard time breathing and needed to be on oxygen for a short amount of time. The NICU team brought him to see me for a brief minute, but I was unable to hold him or touch him before he was gone.

It was almost two hours before I was wheeled on my bed into the NICU to hold my baby. It was over 4 hours before I could walk to the NICU and hold my baby for as long as I wanted and try to breastfeed. My son Easton was born six weeks early on July 4th, 2023, via emergency C-Section.

Reflecting on the birth of my son, I mourn the loss of my ability to have a natural birth. I am constantly thinking, what if, if I only, if I knew. My husband and I have decided this is our last child as I do not want to have another C-Section, and doing a vaginal delivery after C-Section can be very risky. I am telling you this because if things do not go as planned, that is okay. But if things do take a turn for the worse, it is OK to mourn. It is OK to take a little time to acknowledge that you did not get to have that experience. You did something some people only dream of. You created life!

Remember, all deliveries are different, and your experiences may change. Expecting the "perfect birth" might leave you feeling like a failure if things don't go exactly as planned. Planning to have an empowered birth can mean having the support around you that you know and trust and being able to ask questions and make informed decisions. If you decide to have a birth plan, think of it more as a wish list. All childbirths are unpredictable and can change at the drop of a hat. Knowledge is the strongest form of power and acknowledging that the ultimate goal is 100% achievable: a healthy mother and child.

7

Conclusion

Thank you for reading my first book. I hope that the information you received has given you the knowledge and confidence you need to navigate the process of labor and delivery with ease. Remember, you were made for this and have the strength within you to bring your baby into the world safely.

If you enjoyed reading this book, please consider leaving a positive review on Amazon.

8

Resources

Natural Childbirth. (2022, April). Kidshealth.org. Retrieved April 8, 2024, from https://kidshealth.org/en/parents/natural-childbirth.html

Geddes, J. K., & Geddes, J. K. (2023, May 18). Walking during pregnancy. What to Expect. https://www.whattoexpect.com/pregnancy/keeping-fit/week-38/walk-it-off.aspx

foralifethyme@gmail.com. (2024, February 8). Optimizing labor: The role of evening primrose oil in pregnancy. For a Life Thyme LLC. https://foralifethyme.com/evening-primrose-oil-in-pregnancy-natural-labor-induction/

Marcin, A. (2023, July 7). How to do a perineal massage during pregnancy. Healthline. https://www.healthline.com/health/pregnancy/perineal-massage#best-oils

Schulte, L. (2023, November 15). Valuing your body and instincts during birth - Institute for Birth Healing Courses. Institute for Birth Healing

Courses. https://instituteforbirthhealing.com/valuing-your-body-and
-instincts-during-birth/

The circuit. (n.d.). The Miles Circuit. https://www.milescircuit.com/t
he-circuit.html

Counter Pressure Science 3 techniques – MamasteFit. (n.d.). https://m
amastefit.com/counter-pressure-science-3-techniques/

Benefits of a birthing ball | In all stages of birth. (n.d.). The Birth Ball.
https://thebirthball.com/pages/benefits-of-a-birthing-ball

Clinic, C. (2024, April 12). Natural birth: Coping skills for labor without
medication. Cleveland Clinic. https://health.clevelandclinic.org/natur
al-birth

Jacobs, S. (2021, September 1). Avoiding disappointment: How to have
a truly Empowered Birth - Urban Hatch. Urban Hatch. https://www.u
rban-hatch.com/avoiding-disappointment-how-to-have-a-truly-emp
owered-birth/